Table of Contents

Fatty liver is also known as hepatic steatosis. It happens when fat builds up in the liver. Having small amounts of fat in your liver is normal, but too much can become a health problem.

Your liver is the second-largest organ in your body. It helps process nutrients from food and drinks, and filters harmful substances from your blood.

Too much fat in your liver can cause liver inflammation, which can damage your liver and create scarring. In severe cases, this scarring can lead to liver failure.

When fatty liver develops in someone who drinks a lot of alcohol, it's known as alcoholic fatty liver disease (AFLD).

In someone who doesn't drink a lot of alcohol, it's known as nonalcoholic fatty liver disease (NAFLD).

According to a 2017 research review, NAFLD affects up to 25 to 30 percent of peopleTrusted Source in the United States and Europe.

BREAKFAST

1. Crunchwrap

Prep Time: 10 Minutes

Cook Time: 35 Minutes

Servings: 4

Ingredients

Hashbrowns:

- 1 lb. hashbrown potatoes
- 1/4 cup oil for frying
- 1 tablespoon of taco seasoning, Southwestern spices, or Cajun spices
- salt to taste

Crunchwraps

- 1/2 lb. ground pork sausage
- 6 eggs, beaten

- 7 oz. shredded V&V Supremo Chihuahua Brand Quesadilla Cheese (love this for smooth and creamy melting!)
- 5 burrito-sized flour tortillas

Instructions

1. Hashbrowns: Heat the oil over medium heat in a large, wide skillet. Working in batches, add hashbrown potatoes in a thin layer, dust with some spices, and press them gently with a spatula. Cook until golden brown and crispy. Flip and repeat. Remove in chunks with a spatula and transfer to a paper towel lined plate. Season with salt.
2. Sausage and Eggs: Brown the sausage in a large nonstick skillet. When the sausage is cooked, drain off excess oil. Turn the heat down. Add the eggs to the hot pan with the sausage and gently stir around with a spatula until just barely set.
3. Tortilla Pieces: Lay a large tortilla on a flat surface. Cut into fourths (you'll use these as a filler piece).
4. Crunchwrap Time: Layer hashbrowns, sausage and egg mixture, and your V&V Supremo Chihuahua Brand Quesadilla Cheese. Place a filler piece of tortilla

over the top and fold the edges of the tortilla inwards, one section at a time. It will kind of make a star shape (watch the video for a demo). Place in a hot oiled skillet. Cook for a few minutes on each side until the exterior is firm, crunchy, and golden brown. Cut and serve!

Prep Time: 10 Minutes

Cook Time: 20 Minutes

Servings: 2

Ingredients

- 3/4 cup milk
- 2 tablespoons white vinegar
- 1 cup flour
- 2 tablespoons sugar
- 1 teaspoon baking powder
- 1/2 teaspoon baking soda
- 1/2 teaspoon salt
- 1 egg
- 2 tablespoons melted butter
- 1+ cup fresh blueberries
- more butter for the pan

Instructions

1. Mix the milk and vinegar and let it sit for a minute or two (you're making "buttermilk" here).

2. Whisk the dry ingredients together. Whisk the egg, milk, and melted butter into the dry ingredients until just combined.

3. Heat a nonstick pan over medium heat. Melt a little smear of butter in the pan (essential for giving a yummy golden brown crust).

4. Pour about 1/3 cup of batter into the hot skillet and spread it flat-like (it will be pretty thick). Arrange a few blueberries on top. Cook until you see little bubbles on top and the edges starting to firm up. Flip and cook for another 1-2 minutes until the pancakes are sky-high fluffy and cooked through.

5. Serve with butter and maple syrup. But honestly, sometimes I just like to eat these plain.

Prep Time: 10 Minutes

Cook Time: 20 Minutes

Servings: 3-4

Ingredients

- Egg Waffles
- 4 eggs
- 1 1/2 cups frozen hashbrowns (or just a grated potato works, too)
- 1/4 cup bacon or pancetta or cooked sausage (optional)
- 1/4 cup shredded cheese
- a few shakes of garlic powder
- 1/2 – 1 teaspoon salt
- 1/2 cup spinach, torn or cut into small pieces (optional)
- a couple little pieces of cheddar cheese to put on top (for extra cheesy-golden-brown spots)
- Egg Waffle Toppings
- goat cheese
- peppers and garlic confit

- avocado

- romesco sauce (store-bought or homemade)

- chives

- hot sauce!

Instructions

1. Mix the base ingredients together for your egg waffles.

2. Pour about 1/2-3/4 cup onto a nonstick waffle maker (depending on the size of yours). I usually spray mine with cooking spray, but that isn't always necessary if the nonstick is really good.

3. Place the cheese chunks on top and put the lid down. When the light goes off to signal that it's done, check that the eggs are cooked, veggies are soft, and cheese is golden on top. Remove carefully to a plate. (Mine is usually golden with soft veggies in just 1-2 minutes, but if yours isn't done yet, just flip it or give it another minute.)

4. Top with all your toppings! I like goat cheese and pepper and garlic confit, romesco, avocado, and chives, and lots of salt and pepper. My little girls like ketchup. We all win!

Prep Time: 30 Minutes

Cook Time: 40 Minutes

Servings: 6-8

Ingredients

- Green Chile Sausage Gravy
- 1 lb. Appleton Farms Premium Pork Sausage
- 4 tablespoons butter
- 4 tablespoons flour
- 2 cups Simply Nature Organic Whole Milk
- 1/2 teaspoon salt
- 1 can Pueblo Lindo Chopped Green Chiles
- Egg Bake
- 8 Simply Nature Organic Cage Free Eggs
- 1/2 cup Simply Nature Organic Whole Milk
- 1/2 teaspoon salt
- 12-ounce tube of Bake House Creations Jumbo Buttermilk Biscuits (about 6–8 biscuits), cut into small cubes
- 1 cup Happy Farms Shredded Mild Cheddar Cheese

Instructions

1. Cook the Sausage: Brown the sausage in a large cast iron skillet. Remove from pan. Drain off excess grease.

2. Make the Gravy: Melt butter in the same cast iron skillet over medium-low heat. Whisk in flour; stir until thickened, 2-3 minutes. Whisk in the milk, about 1/2 cup at a time, until a smooth gravy comes together. Add salt, diced green chiles, and sausage back to the gravy. Stir to combine.

3. Whisk the Eggs: In a separate bowl, whisk eggs with milk and salt.

4. Assemble the Egg Bake: Preheat the oven to 350 degrees. Place half of the biscuits over the bottom of a greased 9×13 pan. Pour eggs over top. Sprinkle with cheese and dollop with some of the gravy (but save some gravy for later). Arrange with remaining biscuits. Bake for 35 minutes, until eggs are set.

5. Eat Up: Serve slices warm from the oven, with a scoop of that green chile sausage gravy over the top (thin it out with a little more milk so it's semi-pourable, since it usually thickens as it cools). Brunch dreams realized.

Prep Time: 20 Minutes

Cook Time: 30 Minutes

Servings: 14-15

Ingredients

- 2 1/3 cups old-fashioned oats
- 1/2 cup uncooked quinoa
- 1 cup raw nuts (a mix of whole almonds and pecan halves is my favorite)
- 1/2 cup unsweetened shredded coconut
- 1/4 cup chia seeds
- 2 teaspoons ground cinnamon
- 1/2 teaspoon kosher salt
- 1/3 cup pure maple syrup
- 3 tablespoons melted coconut oil or canola oil
- 3 tablespoons unsulphured molasses (not blackstrap)
- 2 teaspoons pure vanilla extract
- 1 large egg white
- 3/4 cup mix-ins of choice: chocolate chips, dried fruit, chopped if larger than a nickel

Instructions

1. Place a rack in the center of your oven and preheat to 300 degrees F. Line a large rimmed baking sheet with parchment paper.

2. In a large bowl, stir together the oats, quinoa, nuts, coconut, chia seeds, cinnamon, and salt with a rubber spatula until combined. Pour in the maple syrup, oil, molasses, and vanilla. Stir to coat, until the dry ingredients are evenly moistened.

3. In a small bowl, briskly whisk the egg white with a fork or small whisk until it is foamy. Add it to the granola mixture and stir, doing your best to evenly incorporate the egg white throughout.

4. Carefully pour the granola onto the prepared baking sheet and spread into a single layer, pressing it down with the back of the spatula. Bake for 20 minutes, then remove the granola from the oven. With a large, flexible spatula, carefully flip large sections of the granola over, doing your best to keep them intact. With the back of the spatula, press the granola back into a single layer. Rotate the pan 180 degrees, return it to the oven, then bake for an additional 15 to 20 minutes, until the granola is golden brown, feels

almost dry to the touch, and smells irresistible. It will continue to crisp as it cools.

5. Place the baking sheet on a cooling rack. Let the granola cool completely on the sheet (no cheating!), then carefully stir in the mix- ins, breaking up the granola as you do. Enjoy with milk, yogurt, overnight oats, over ice cream or frozen yogurt, or on its own by the handful.

Prep Time: 20 Minutes

Cook Time: 15 Minutes

Servings: 12-15

Ingredients

Streusel:

- 1/4 cup butter
- 1/2 cup brown sugar
- 1/2 cup flour
- pinch of salt

Cheesecake Layer:

- 6 ounces cream cheese
- 1 egg yolk
- 1/4 cup sugar
- Triple Berry Muffins:
- 1/2 cup butter, softened
- 1/2 cup granulated sugar
- 1/4 cup brown sugar
- 2 eggs
- 1/2 cup plain yogurt

- 1 tablespoon vanilla extract

- 1 3/4 cups flour

- 1 teaspoon baking soda

- 1 teaspoon baking powder

- 1/2 teaspoon salt

- 1 heaping cup of a frozen berry blend (raspberries, blueberries, and blackberries) – not thawed

Instructions

1. Streusel: Soften or melt the butter, and use your hands to mix it with the brown sugar, flour, and salt. You should get the consistency that matches the pictures above – like small pebbles.

2. Cheesecake Layer: Beat the cream cheese until smooth. Add egg and sugar; beat again until smooth.

3. Muffins: Preheat the oven to 425 degrees. Beat the butter and sugars together until creamed. Add the eggs, yogurt, and vanilla; stir until combined. Add the flour, baking soda, baking powder, and salt; mix until just combined. The batter will be thick. Fold in the frozen berries just before assembling the muffins.

4. Layering: Line a muffin tin with paper liners. Press 1-2 tablespoons of batter into the bottom of each muffin

tin. Flatten with the back of a wet spoon. Pour a spoonful of cheesecake mixture over the top. Cover with another 1-2 tablespoons of muffin batter. Sprinkle with streusel.

5. Bake: Bake for 5 minutes at 425 degrees, then turn the oven temperature down to 350 and bake for another 15-18 minutes. Voila! Look at those beauties! You did it!

Prep Time: 20 Minutes

Cook Time: 10 Minutes

Servings: 3-4

Ingredients

Egg Waffles:

- 4 eggs
- 1 1/2 cups frozen hashbrowns (or just a grated potato works, too)
- 1/4 cup bacon or pancetta or cooked sausage (optional)
- 1/4 cup shredded cheese
- a few shakes of garlic powder
- 1/2 – 1 teaspoon salt
- 1/2 cup spinach, torn or cut into small pieces (optional)
- a couple little pieces of cheddar cheese to put on top (for extra cheesy-golden-brown spots)

Egg Waffle Toppings:

- goat cheese

- peppers and garlic confit

- avocado

- romesco sauce (store-bought or homemade)

- chives

- hot sauce!

Instructions

1. Mix the base ingredients together for your egg waffles.

2. Pour about 1/2-3/4 cup onto a nonstick waffle maker (depending on the size of yours). I usually spray mine with cooking spray, but that isn't always necessary if the nonstick is really good.

3. Place the cheese chunks on top and put the lid down. When the light goes off to signal that it's done, check that the eggs are cooked, veggies are soft, and cheese is golden on top. Remove carefully to a plate. (Mine is usually golden with soft veggies in just 1-2 minutes, but if yours isn't done yet, just flip it or give it another minute.)

4. Top with all your toppings! I like goat cheese and pepper and garlic confit, romesco, avocado, and chives, and lots of salt and pepper. My little girls like ketchup. We all win!

Prep Time: 20 Minutes

Cook Time: 20 Minutes

Servings: 3-4

Ingredients

Crispy Tofu:

- 1 block of extra firm tofu
- 2 tablespoons cornstarch
- 1 tablespoon soy sauce
- 2 tablespoons olive oil
- Apricot Sauce:
- 1/3 cup apricot preserves
- 1 tablespoons soy sauce
- 1–2 tablespoons rice vinegar
- 1/2 teaspoon each cumin, paprika, and onion powder
- 1–2 cloves garlic, grated (2 for more garlic flavor, obviously)
- 1/4 teaspoon salt (more to taste)

Extras for Serving:

- toasted sesame oil to taste (I like about 1-2 tablespoons)
- chives and/or cilantro for topping
- steamed green beans
- cooked rice

Instructions

1. Cut the tofu block in half horizontally (like a hamburger). If using extra firm high protein tofu, it helps to cut it in half again horizontally. Press the water out of the tofu by wrapping it in paper towels and setting a few heavy books on top of it. Let it stay like that for a few minutes while you prep the sauce.
2. Whisk the sauce ingredients together.
3. Take each piece of tofu and gently pull it into small chunks with your hands (this just gives the tofu pieces a unique shape and texture that holds onto the sauce really well). Place the chunks in a bowl. Toss with soy sauce and a teaspoon or two of olive oil; then sprinkle with cornstarch and give it a few gentle tosses to coat.
4. In a nonstick skillet over medium high heat, heat the olive oil and then add the cornstarched tofu. Leave it undisturbed for a few minutes on each side, letting it

get really nice and brown and crispy – this can take 10-15 minutes. Flip and repeat until the whole batch is browned and crispy.

5. While it's browning, you can start up your rice and/or sides!

6. Finally, add the sauce to the tofu and remove from heat – the pan will still be hot, so it'll be sizzly and smell really good from the garlic. The sauce will coat the tofu right away. heart eyes

7. Top with the green onions and/or cilantro, sesame seeds, and sesame oil. Serve with rice and green beans, and finish with more salt and lots of black pepper to taste. The tender crunch of the beans with the steamy rice and sticky tofu! SO good.

Prep Time: 20 Minutes

Cook Time: 50 Minutes

Servings: 12

Ingredients

- 1 tablespoon butter
- 1 shallot, minced
- 2 cups veggies – I used mushrooms, asparagus, and spinach
- 8 Simply Nature Organic Grade A Cage Free Eggs
- 1 1/4 cup heavy cream
- 1 cup Emporium Selection Specialty Shredded Gouda Cheese
- 1 teaspoon salt (more to taste)
- 2 unbaked Bakehouse Creations Pie Crust

Instructions

1. Melt the butter over medium high heat. Add the mushrooms; sauté until browned and soft. Add the shallots; sauté until fragrant. Add asparagus; sauté

until softened and bright green. Season with a pinch of salt.

2. Whisk eggs and heavy cream together. Add cooked veggies, cheese, and salt.

3. Press pie crust into a 10-inch pie pan and gently crimp the edges so they look nice. (This recipe is enough for two quiches, so just do this twice if you're making both at the same time.)

4. Preheat the oven to 350 degrees. Poke tiny holes in the bottom of the crust with a fork. Bake the pie crust for 10 minutes, until partially baked.

5. Pour the egg and veggie mixture into the pie dish (stop when you start to get to the top of the pie edges). Bake for 15 minutes.

6. Remove pan from oven and cover the pie edges with a foil crown so the edges don't overbrown. Bake for another 15 minutes.

7. Slice and serve! Serve with a little spring mix salad, fruit, or muffins for brunch goals. Yum.

Prep Time: 55 Minutes

Cook Time: 6hrs Minutes

Servings: 8

Ingredients

- 3 cups all-purpose flour (405 grams or 14.3 ounces)
- 1 1/2 teaspoons salt
- 1/2 teaspoon instant yeast
- 1 1/2 cups room temperature water

Instructions

Dough Prep:

1. In a large mixing bowl, whisk the flour, salt, and yeast together until mixed. Stir in the water until a chunky, thick dough forms. If it needs a little more water, add a few more tablespoons, just enough to get it barely wet throughout. It's gonna look scrappy and weird and you're going to question me on whether or not this will work, but it will. Cover the mixing bowl with

plastic wrap and let it rest for 12-18 hours at room temperature. Overnight is ideal here, kids.

Prep For Baking:

2. When you're ready to bake, preheat the oven to 450. Stick a 6 quart enamel coated cast iron Lodge Dutch Oven (or similar) in the oven for about 30 minutes to heat. At this point, the dough should be big and puffy and pretty loose, with little bubbles in it. Gently scrape the dough out onto a well-floured surface. (Remember: NO KNEAD.) Gently shape it into a ball with flour on the outside, set on a piece of parchment, and cover with plastic while your pan heats up.

Bake:

3. Remove the plastic from the dough. Lift the dough and parchment together into the pan so the parchment lines the bottom of the hot pan (be careful not to touch the pan since it's very hot). Bake, covered, for 30 minutes. Remove the cover and bake another 10-15 minutes to get the exterior nice and golden brown and crispy. Voila! Done. Miracle no-knead bread, you boss you.

11. Chipotle Orange Shrimp with Cilantro Rice

Prep Time: 15 Minutes

Cook Time: 25 Minutes

Servings: 2-4

Ingredients

Chipotle Orange Sauce:

- 1 chipotle pepper (or half of one pepper, for a less spicy version)
- 3/4 cup heavy cream
- 2 cloves garlic
- 1/2 teaspoon salt
- zest of one orange

Shrimp and Rice:

- a drizzle of olive oil
- 1 pound uncooked shrimp, tails removed, patted dry
- 1/2 teaspoon cumin
- 1 1/2 cups white rice (I like jasmine rice or just plain long grain rice)

- a big handful of chopped cilantro
- optional, for serving: zippy cucumbers (see notes)

Instructions

4. Sauce: Blend sauce ingredients together until mostly smooth. But don't overblend! See notes.
5. Rice: Cook rice according to package directions. Stir in cilantro and salt to taste (+ add lime juice, or the juice of the zested orange, if you want some citrus goodness in there).
6. Shrimp: Heat the oil over medium high heat. Add the shrimp and sauté for 2 minutes on each side, sprinkling with the cumin, plus some salt and pepper.
7. Finish: Add the sauce and simmer for another 5 minutes or so. Serve shrimp over rice, with a salad or some fresh zippy cucumbers.

Prep Time: 15 Minutes

Cook Time: 10 Minutes

Servings: 4

Ingredients

- 2 tablespoons DeLallo Private Reserve Extra Virgin Olive Oil
- 4 cloves garlic, thinly sliced or minced
- 1/4 cup DeLallo Tomato Paste
- 1/2 teaspoon Italian seasoning
- 4 cups chicken broth
- salt to taste
- 1 cup DeLallo Orzo Pasta
- 2 cups chopped or shredded cooked chicken (I use the pulled meat from a rotisserie chicken)
- 1/4 cup heavy cream
- 1–2 cups water as desired
- parmesan, herbs, red pepper flakes, and lemon for serving
- bread for serving
- pesto for serving (optional)

Instructions

1. Heat the olive oil in a soup pot over medium high heat. (See notes on types of pan to use!) Add the garlic; sauté for 1-2 minutes until soft and fragrant but not browned.

2. Add the tomato paste and Italian seasoning; cook until it becomes caramelized and turns a deep red color, about 5 minutes.

3. Add the broth gradually until the mixture incorporates into a smooth liquid. This is a good time to add salt; I recommend tasting the liquid to see how much salt it needs depending on how salty your broth was. Otherwise just add 1/2 teaspoon to start, and add from there.

4. Add the orzo and bring the whole thing to a simmer for about 10 minutes until the orzo is soft. If needed, add a cup more of water and/or broth to get your desired consistency. Stir in heavy cream.

5. Add the chicken and squeeze in a bunch of lemon juice to wake the whole thing up.

6. Serve topped with Parmesan, herbs, red pepper flakes, and hot crusty bread. If you want, serve with a little side of pesto for dipping the bread in before dunking in the soup. YUM. So good!

Prep Time: 15 Minutes

Cook Time: 20 Minutes

Servings: 4-5

Ingredients

Pasta and Meatballs:

- 1–2 tablespoons olive oil (2 especially if your sauce doesn't have much oil it in)
- 1/2 to 1lb. frozen chicken meatballs (or other pre-made meatballs – I used ones that were already cooked) – about 2 cups if you're eyeballing
- one 32-ounce jar of your favorite tomato pasta sauce
- 1 cup chicken broth
- 1 1/2 cups small pasta – I like to use ditalini
- salt and pepper to taste

Herbed Lemon Ricotta

- 1 pound fresh ricotta – mascarpone is a bit more creamy / melty and also delicious!
- juice of 1 lemon + a little bit of zest
- 1 garlic clove, finely grated

- 1/4 cup olive oil
- 1 cup finely chopped mixed chives, parsley, basil
- Salt and pepper to taste

Instructions

1. Place meatballs in the Instant Pot; drizzle with olive oil. Sauté for a couple minutes to get the meatballs a bit browned on the outside – they don't need to be fully thawed.
2. Add in this order: pasta, sauce, chicken broth. Do not stir. Cook on high pressure for 3 minutes.
3. Release steam right away (so your pasta doesn't overcook and get mushy). Stir to incorporate. A small amount of sticking is normal, but with a few gentle stirs it will lift up and come together perfectly. It will be saucy at first; if you let it rest a few minutes, the sauce will absorb into the pasta and it'll get a little less saucy. It's delicious to eat either way!
4. Mix your herbed ricotta ingredients together while the pasta cooks.
5. Serve the hot pasta in bowls with dollops of the ricotta over the top.

Prep Time: 15 Minutes

Cook Time: 25 Minutes

Servings: 4-6

Ingredients

Meatballs and Such:

- one 22-ounce bag of store-bought frozen meatballs (or homemade, if you've got them / got the time)
- 2 bell peppers (yellow and red), sliced
- 1–2 zucchini, sliced into half moons
- 2 tablespoons harissa paste
- olive oil, garlic powder, lemon juice, salt

Whipped Feta:

- one 6-ounce container feta cheese
- 1–2 ounces cream cheese or sour cream or I've used plain yogurt in a pinch
- 1 clove garlic
- Extras:
- hummus
- pita

- olives / lemon wedges

Instructions

1. Sheet Pan, Part One: Preheat the oven to 425 degrees. Place the peppers on one side of a large sheet pan. Drizzle with oil and sprinkle with salt. Mix the harissa with a little bit of olive oil, lemon juice, and garlic powder until you have a nice spreadable red paste. Coat your meatballs with the sauce (you can do this by tossing the meatballs in a bowl with the sauce if they're pre-cooked, or just brushing the meatballs directly on the sheet pan if your meatballs are raw). Add meatballs to the center of the sheet pan. Bake for 15-20 minutes.

2. Sheet Pan, Part Two: Add the zucchini to the pan with some olive oil and salt. Roast for another 10 minutes. For extra browning on everything, broil for about 5 minutes.

3. Whip That Feta: In a food processor, chopper, or blender, whip up the feta, cream cheese, and garlic until a thick and creamy sauce forms.

4. Serve: Serve meatballs and veggies with a dollop of hummus, your whipped feta, pita wedges, and

anything else you like (olives, lemon, etc.). And now DEVOUR. And repeat. And repeat. And repeat.

Prep Time: 15 Minutes

Cook Time: 15 Minutes

Servings: 4

Ingredients

Pork:

- 1/4 to 1/2 cup teriyaki sauce (I like the SoyVay brand!)
- 1 pound thinly sliced pork tenderloin (you can buy this pre-cut at a lot of stores, sometimes labeled as "stir fry")
- 1–2 cups fresh pineapple chunks
- olive oil for sautéing

Rice:

- one 14-ounce can full fat coconut milk
- 1 1/2 cups water
- 2 cups jasmine rice

Toppings:

- lime zest
- cilantro

- thinly sliced jalapeño
- crunchy onions

Instructions

1. Prep: Marinate the pork with 1/4 cup of the sauce for 2-3 hours, or a full day. This is low-key and low-stress. Just do it whenever you think of it.
2. Rice: Add the rice ingredients to an Instant Pot. Cook on high pressure for 3 minutes, followed by a natural pressure release for 10-15 minutes (just let it sit there). Release the steam, fluff with a fork, season with a little salt, and attempt not to eat the whole thing.
3. Pork: Heat a tablespoon of olive oil in a nonstick skillet or grill pan over medium high heat. Add *just* the pork, discarding the excess sauce – if you add all the sauce with it, it will steam the pork instead of caramelizing it. Leave the pork undisturbed in the hot pan for a few minutes at a time to get better caramelization. Throw the pineapple in there and let it get saucy and caramelized, too. Add a few additional tablespoons of sauce AFTER you've gotten it nice and brown.

4. Serve: Top your luscious rice with a scoop of the saucy pineapple pork and finish with lime zest, cilantro, crunchy onions, and little slices of jalapeño.

Prep Time: 20 Minutes

Cook Time: 20 Minutes

Servings: 4

Ingredients

For the Chicken:

- 1 lb. Simply Nature Organic Thin Sliced Chicken Breast Fillets, pounded or cut in half lengthwise so they are flat and thin
- 1/4 cup Burman's Hot Sauce
- 2 tablespoons Specially Selected Raw Honey
- 1 teaspoon garlic powder
- 1 teaspoon paprika
- 1 teaspoon salt
- 1/2 teaspoon onion powder
- black pepper to taste

For the Rice:

- 1 cup Simply Nature Organic White Rice
- 1 package Season's Choice Riced Cauliflower

- 1–2 tablespoons of Simply Nature Organic Extra Virgin Olive Oil
- salt to taste

For the Cucumber Salad:

- cucumbers, sliced
- cherry tomatoes, halved
- Park Street Deli Dill Dip or avocado cilantro dressing

Instructions

1. Marinate Chicken: Place chicken, buffalo sauce, honey, garlic powder, paprika, salt, onion powder, and black pepper in a bowl or bag. Place in the fridge to marinate for 30 minutes to 2 hours.
2. Cook Rice: Cook rice according to package directions.
3. Roast Cauliflower: Place cauliflower rice on a sheet pan. Drizzle with olive oil and sprinkle with salt. Roast at 425 degrees for 20-30 minutes until partially browned and a little roasty. Add roasted cauliflower rice to cooked rice. (Optional: season with garlic powder, lemon juice, parsley, or parmesan.)
4. Cook Chicken: Heat a grill pan over high heat. Add a little olive oil if needed, then add the marinated

chicken pieces, discarding extra marinade. Cook for a few minutes on each side until nice and browned, and no longer pink on the inside. Remove from the pan and let rest for a few minutes.

5. Serve: Slice chicken and serve with a scoop of cauliflower rice. Top with sliced cucumber and tomato and a dollop of dill dip or ranch dressing.

Prep Time: 10 Minutes

Cook Time: 20 Minutes

Servings: 4

Ingredients

Ginger Peanut Chicken:

- 1 1/4 pounds chicken thighs, fat trimmed, cut into small bite-sized pieces
- 1-inch piece of ginger, grated
- 3 green onions, thinly sliced (white parts and green parts separated)
- zest and juice of 1-2 limes
- 2 tablespoons brown sugar
- 1 1/2 teaspoons salt
- 1 tablespoon olive oil or avocado oil
- 2–3 cloves garlic, minced
- 1/2 cup chopped roasted peanuts
- 1/2 cup chopped cilantro
- spinach, bok choy, etc.
- Coconut Rice

- 2 cups white or jasmine rice
- 1 1/2 cups water
- 1 can coconut milk
- a pinch of salt

Instructions

1. Marinate Chicken: In a stainless steel bowl, mix the chicken with the ginger, green onions (white parts), lime zest, brown sugar, salt, and oil. Marinate for 20 minutes-2 hours.

2. Rice: Add the rice ingredients to an Instant Pot. Cook on high pressure for 3 minutes, followed by a natural pressure release for 10-15 minutes (it won't be quite done yet after 3 minutes – it needs the rest time to finish cooking). Release the steam, fluff with a fork, and attempt not to eat the whole thing! (Don't have an Instant Pot? Alternative methods are in the notes section!)

3. Cook Chicken: Heat a large skillet (nonstick or cast iron work well) to medium-high heat. Add the marinated chicken to the pan, working in 1-2 batches depending on the size of your pan. Leave the chicken

sitting undisturbed for several minutes to get a nice caramelization on the chicken.

4. Adding Extras: When all the chicken is cooked, turn the heat down slightly and add the peanuts and garlic to the pan. Sauté for 3-5 minutes to get the peanuts roasty and the garlic nice and fragrant.

5. Finish by adding in the cilantro, green onion, and spinach. Squeeze lime juice into the pan and season with more salt and pepper as needed.

6. Serve over coconut rice! SO simple but so good.

Prep Time: 10 Minutes

Cook Time: 50 Minutes

Servings: 4-8

Ingredients

- 4 ounces diced pancetta
- 1 lb. ground sausage
- 1 small yellow onion, diced
- 6 cloves garlic, minced
- 2 tablespoons tomato paste
- 2 28–ounce cans whole peeled tomatoes (I like San Marzano tomatoes), crushed by hand
- 1 teaspoon salt
- 1 teaspoon fresh oregano, minced
- 1 teaspoon red pepper flakes
- 1–2 cups chicken broth or water to thin the sauce
- 2–4 tablespoons butter to tame the heat (if you want)
- 1 cup sliced pepperoncini (more to taste)
- bucatini pasta for serving
- pecorino cheese for topping

Instructions

1. In a large heavy pot like a Dutch oven, cook the pancetta over medium high heat until very, very browned. You want them to be well-done; browned, almost crispy, and concentrated with flavor. Remove pancetta and set aside; drain oil out of the pan.

2. In the same pot, brown the Italian sausage until cooked through and crumbled. Remove sausage and set aside, saving a little bit of the oil in the pan.

3. In the same pot, add the onion and garlic. (Add a bit of olive oil if needed.) Sauté until soft and fragrant. Add tomato paste and sauté for another 2-3 minutes.

4. Add crushed tomatoes, salt, oregano, and red pepper flakes. Add sausage and pancetta back in to the pot. Cover and simmer for 30 minutes.

5. Add the broth until desired consistency is reached. Add butter if you want.

6. Add pepperoncini. Simmer for 5 more minutes until the pepperoncini are very soft but not broken down.

7. Cook bucatini according to package directions; drain and return to pot. Pour sauce over cooked bucatini and keep over heat for a few minutes to help the sauce and noodles come together.

8. Top bucatini with pecorino cheese. What a moment.

Prep Time: 10 Minutes

Cook Time: 10 Minutes

Servings: 4-5

Ingredients

Lettuce Wraps:

- olive oil
- One 14-ounce block extra firm tofu – minimally pressed to remove water
- about 2 cups cooked brown rice and/or quinoa or other grains – I use the 8.5 ounce precooked packages so it's very, very easy
- butter lettuce or leaf lettuce for wrapping
- spicy mayo (see notes)
- chopped peanuts or crispy onions for topping
- SOS Peanut Sauce
- 1/2 cup teriyaki sauce
- juice of 1 orange
- 1/4 cup peanut butter
- a squirt of Sriracha or other chile sauce if you want

- If you have a bit more time, you can also use this amazing homemade peanut sauce.

Instructions

1. Cook the tofu: Heat a few swishes of oil in a nonstick skillet over medium high heat. Add the tofu and crumble in the pan. Cook until slightly browned. While that's cooking, whisk up all sauce ingredients in a bowl.
2. Add rice and sauce: Add the rice and most of the sauce to the pan. Sauté for 5 minutes or so – just enough to get some browning / light caramelization and get everything nice and yummy. Season with salt to taste.
3. Fill and serve: Spoon your tofu and brown rice filling into crispy little pieces of lettuce. Top with something crunchy (peanuts? crispy onions?) and something creamy (spicy mayo all the way) and drizzle with a little extra sauce, and now tell me this isn't your favorite meal of the week.

Prep Time: 10 Minutes

Cook Time: 30 Minutes

Servings: 4

Ingredients

Parmesan Risotto:

- 1 tablespoon butter
- 1 clove minced garlic or 1 minced shallot (or both)
- 1 cup DeLallo Risotto Arborio Rice
- 1/2 cup white wine (sub chicken broth + a little lemon juice)
- 3-4 cups of chicken broth
- 1/2 cup Parmesan cheese
- optional: tiny drizzle of truffle oil

Pesto Shrimp:

- 1–2 pounds jumbo shrimp (shells removed and tails on or off, whatever you prefer)
- 2 cloves garlic
- 2 tablespoons olive oil
- 1 teaspoon salt

- zest of 1 lemon (optional)
- 1/4 cup DeLallo jarred pesto
- 1–2 roma, beefsteak, or any kind of fresh juicy tomatoes, chopped
- herbs for topping

Instructions

1. Marinate the Shrimp: Place the shrimp, garlic, 1 tablespoon olive oil, salt, and lemon zest in a bowl or plastic bag. Mix it all together so the shrimp is coated with all that flavor goodness. Stick it back in the fridge to let it marinate while you make the risotto (for about 1 hour, if you can).

2. Make the Risotto: In a large non-stick skillet over medium heat, melt the butter. Add the garlic or shallots and saute for a minute or two, until soft and fragrant.

3. Add the arborio rice, stir to coat with butter. Add the white wine and enjoy the sizzles. Add the broth, 1/2 cup at a time, and simmer/stir after each addition until the rice is soft and creamy.

4. When the risotto is done, add the Parmesan and stir until incorporated. Add truffle oil if you want (omg it's so good). Salt + pepp to taste.

5. Make the Pesto Shrimp: Heat the remaining 1 tablespoon olive oil in a skillet over medium-high heat (I use nonstick for this). Add the shrimp and cook for 2-3 minutes on each side, depending on their size. Brush the cooked shrimp with the pesto for the last 60 seconds or so of cooking.

6. Serve risotto topped with those juicy pesto shrimp. Speckle some chopped fresh tomatoes around in there and top with herbs or something delicate and green (I used microgreens in the photo). Salt, pepper, a little more lemon juice and you're in a very happy place.

21. Garlic Cream Bucatini with Peas And Asparagus

Prep Time: 10 Minutes

Cook Time: 50 Minutes

Servings: 6

Ingredients

- 1/2 pound of DeLallo Bucatini Pasta
- 2 tablespoons butter
- half a bunch of asparagus, ends trimmed and sliced diagonally (about 1 1/2 cups once cut)
- 4 cloves garlic, grated
- 3/4 cup chicken or vegetable broth
- 1 cup heavy cream
- half of a bag of frozen peas (about a heaping cup)
- zest of one lemon
- lemon juice to taste
- salt and pepper to taste
- some golden crispies aka breadcrumbs for topping

Instructions

1. Cook pasta to al dente according to package directions.

2. Melt butter over medium heat. Add asparagus and cook for 5 minutes, until soft and bright green. (You'll simmer the asparagus a bit longer in the sauce, so it's okay if it's still a little firm.)

3. Add garlic and sauté for 1-2 minutes, until fragrant.

4. Add broth and heavy cream; bring to a low simmer. Once it thickens into more of a sauce, add in the frozen peas for the final few minutes of cooking. Season with the lemon juice, lemon zest, salt, and pepper.

5. Toss the sauce with the pasta; keep it all over low heat for a few minutes so the pasta and the sauce really come together. Let stand for a few minutes if necessary for everything to thicken and the sauce to really cling on to the pasta. Top with lots and lots of breadcrumbs, and some rotisserie chicken or sautéed shrimp if you want! So yum!

Prep Time: 10 Minutes

Cook Time: 40 Minutes

Servings: 6

Ingredients

- 3 tablespoons extra virgin olive oil
- 3 cloves garlic, smashed or thinly sliced
- one 28-ounce can whole peeled San Marzano tomatoes
- 1 teaspoon kosher salt
- Freshly ground black pepper to taste
- 4 cups vegetable or chicken broth
- 1/4 cup packed fresh basil, chopped or torn
- 2–3 cups dry bread, torn or cut into cubes

Instructions

1. Heat the olive oil in a large pot over medium heat. Add the garlic; sauté for 1 minute.

2. In a separate bowl, crush tomatoes by hand. Add them into the pot. Add salt and pepper. Partially cover and simmer over medium heat for about ten minutes.

3. Add the broth and basil; bring back to a simmer for another ten minutes.

4. Add the bread cubes; simmer for another ten minutes until the bread is soft. You can use a potato masher to further break down the bread to your desired texture.

5. Serve with Parmesan cheese, extra olive oil, and more fresh basil! Simplicity and top notch ingredients... it's just stunning.

Prep Time: 10 Minutes

Cook Time: 40 Minutes

Servings: 6

Ingredients

Salad:

- 1 cup Simple Nature Organic Quinoa, uncooked
- 5 ears sweet corn, cut off the cob
- 1 can Simply Nature Organic Black Beans, rinsed
- 1 package mini sweet peppers, sliced into small rings (about 2–3 cups)
- olive oil for cooking
- 1 cup chopped fresh cilantro

Dressing:

- 1/3 cup Burman's Mayonnaise
- 1/4 cup buttermilk
- 1 clove garlic, grated
- 1 teaspoon Stonemill Chili Powder
- 1/2 to 1 teaspoon salt
- juice and zest of two limes

- Pueblo Lindo Grated Cotija Cheese for topping

Instructions

1. Cook quinoa and prep ingredients.

2. Drizzle a generous amount of olive oil in a skillet and add the pepper rings. Cook over medium heat, stirring occasionally, for about 20 minutes or until very soft and roasty-looking. Squeeze a little lime juice in the pan to lift all the browned bits off the bottom of the pan when you're done! More flavor!

3. Whisk up the dressing ingredients. Taste and adjust. It's okay if it's super salty – it's going on a bunch of raw, unseasoned ingredients so we want it to have lots of flavor!

4. Toss ingredients or arrange in a bowl just before serving (quinoa, corn, beans, peppers, cilantro, and topped with dressing and cheese). Serve with grilled chicken, dip with chips, or on its own as a meal!

Prep Time: 10 Minutes

Cook Time: 20 Minutes

Servings: 6

Ingredients

Gochujang Sauce:

- 3 tablespoons soy sauce
- 2–3 tablespoons gochujang sauce
- 2 tablespoons tomato paste
- 2 tablespoons peanut butter
- 2 tablespoons water
- 1–2 tablespoons brown sugar
- 1 tablespoon sesame oil
- 1 clove minced garlic
- 1–2 cups broth or water for thinning the sauce

Noodles:

- 1 pound ground chicken (could also use pork)
- 1/2 teaspoon salt
- freshly ground black pepper
- 2 packets ramen or stir fry noodles (just the noodles)

- a couple big handfuls of fresh spinach
- chives, scallions, cilantro, basil, or whatever herbs you like for topping
- salt, chili oil, or sesame seeds for finishing

Instructions

1. Whisk the sauce ingredients (except the extra broth) in a small bowl or shake together in a jar. It should form a thick sauce.
2. Cook the chicken in a large skillet over medium high heat. Season generously with salt and pepper.
3. Boil the noodles for just a few minutes to soften. Drain and set aside.
4. When the chicken is done, add spinach, cooked noodles, and sauce to the pan, keeping it over medium high heat. Toss to combine; heat until the spinach is wilted. Add extra water or broth to thin the sauce, a little at a time, to get the sauciness that you like (I usually add about 1 1/2 cups total).
5. Serve topped with fresh herbs, scallions, chili oil, sesame seeds, and whatever else you like.

Prep Time: 10 Minutes

Cook Time: 40 Minutes

Servings: 6-8

Ingredients

Red Chile Chicken Tacos:

- 1 pound boneless skinless chicken thighs
- olive oil, salt, and pepper
- 8 oz. of red chile enchilada sauce (I like the Frontera brand pouches)
- one 14–ounce can pinto beans, rinsed and drained

Creamy Corn

- 1/4 cup mayo
- 2 tablespoons cream cheese
- 2 cups frozen or fresh sweet corn
- 1 clove garlic, grated
- 1/2 teaspoon salt
- 1 teaspoon cumin
- 1 teaspoon chili powder
- lime juice to taste

- Pickled Onions

- 1 red onion, thinly sliced

- 1/2 cup red wine vinegar

- 1/2 cup water

- 1 teaspoon salt

- 1 tablespoon sugar

Extras

- corn tortillas (I like to quickly pan-fry mine in a shallow skillet of hot oil to make them extra soft)
- cilantro

Instructions

1. For the pickled onions: Transfer red onion slices to a jar. Add red wine vinegar and water. Add your salt and sugar. Shake a few times and set in the fridge while you make everything else.

2. For the chicken: Heat a skillet over medium-high heat. Add olive oil. Add the chicken and season with salt and pepper. Sauté for 7-10 minutes, or until cooked through. Remove from the heat and shred or cut into smaller pieces. Add chicken pieces back to the pan with the sauce and the beans. Simmer gently until

sauce has thickened and it looks ready to be taco filling.

3. For the corn: Mix all ingredients in a small bowl. Taste and adjust.

4. For the tacos: Fill tortillas with the chicken mixture. Top with the creamy corn and pickled red onions. Finish with cilantro.

Prep Time: 25 Minutes

Cook Time: 1hrs 40 Minutes

Servings: 4-6

Ingredients

The Smoked Ranch:

- 1/2 cup mayo
- 1/2 cup full-fat Greek yogurt or sour cream
- 1/2 cup milk or buttermilk
- 1 teaspoon white vinegar or lemon juice (more to taste)
- 2 teaspoons freeze-dried dill
- 2 teaspoons freeze-dried chives
- 1–2 teaspoons smoked paprika
- 1/2 teaspoon onion powder
- 1/2 teaspoon garlic powder
- 1/2 teaspoon salt
- black pepper to taste
- The Pepper Confit
- 3 tablespoons olive oil

- 1 pound mini sweet peppers, sliced into rings
- 3 cloves garlic, sliced into thin pieces
- 1 tablespoon red wine vinegar
- salt to taste

The You-Picks:

- spinach or salad greens (about 2 cups per serving)
- salmon or chicken (about 3-4 ounces per serving)
- avocado (about half of one avocado per serving)
- bacon, cooked and crumbled
- fire-roasted corn
- sunflower seeds

Instructions

1. Smoked Ranch: Shake all ingredients in a jar until smooth. Taste and adjust. Make it yours!
2. Pepper Confit: Heat the olive oil in a skillet over medium heat. Add the peppers and sauté until brown and very soft, stirring only occasionally so you get some nice browning on them. I usually cook them for 20-30 minutes. During the last 10-15 minutes, add in the garlic with the peppers to get it nice and golden and soft (just make sure you don't burn it). During the

last 5 minutes, add the vinegar to add some zip and pull up any browned bits from the bottom of the pan.

3. Bacon: Bake at 400 degrees for 20 minutes. Drain and cool on a paper-towel lined plate. Crumble for the salad.

4. Salmon: Pat dry and season with salt and pepper. Bake at 400 degrees for 8-10 minutes (depending on the size of your piece of salmon and desired doneness).

5. Salad: Assemble everything over greens and drizzle with the smoked ranch. SO GOOD.

Prep Time: 25 Minutes

Cook Time: 50 Minutes

Servings: 4

Ingredients

Zaalouk:

- 1 eggplant
- olive oil and salt
- one 14-ounce can crushed tomatoes (I used crushed San Marzano tomatoes)
- 6 cloves garlic
- 2 teaspoons paprika
- 2 teaspoons cumin
- 1/2 cup fresh parsley
- red pepper flakes for heat (optional)
- 1 teaspoon salt (more to taste)
- Toast, etc.:
- sourdough or Tuscan style sliced bread
- a generous amount of olive oil
- fresh burrata

- olive oil, salt, pepper, and more herbs for topping

Instructions

1. Preheat the oven to 400 degrees.
2. Cut the eggplant in half lengthwise. Make small cuts that allow you to tuck the garlic cloves into the eggplant so they are almost completely inside (so you can roast them without burning them).
3. Drizzle the halves with olive oil and salt; roast for 30-45 minutes until the eggplant is super soft and pulls away from the skin easily.
4. Transfer the eggplant and roasted garlic to a small saucepan; add tomatoes and spices. Mash with a potato masher or the back of a wooden spoon until you get a chunky-but-smooth-ish texture.
5. Simmer for 15 minutes or so. Add the parsley and season to taste.
6. For the grilled bread, heat a skillet over medium heat. Add a generous couple swizzles of olive oil (probably 2 tablespoons or so) and add your sliced bread to the pan. Cook until golden brown and toasty on both sides.

7. To serve, top your toasts with a smear of zaalouk and
    a hunk of fresh burrata. Top with olive oil, herbs, salt
    and pepper.

Prep Time: 25 Minutes

Cook Time: 1hrs 10 Minutes

Servings: 8

Ingredients

- 2 pounds green beans
- 2 tablespoons butter
- 1 shallot, thinly sliced
- 2 tablespoons all-purpose flour
- 1/4 cup white wine
- 3/4 cup whole milk
- 1 cup vegetable broth
- 2 teaspoons soy sauce
- 1 garlic clove, grated
- 1/2 cup shredded gruyere
- 1 teaspoon salt
- 1 cup crispy fried onions

Instructions

1. Preheat the oven to 375 degrees. Bring a large pot of water to a boil. Working in two batches, blanch the green beans until they're bright green and tender-crisp, about 1-2 minutes. Drain the green beans and transfer them to a casserole dish.

2. Melt the butter in a saucepan over medium heat. Add in the shallot, cooking for a couple minutes until tender. Whisk in the flour, and cook for a couple minutes until the mixture is golden brown. Slowly add in the wine, broth, soy sauce, and milk – separately, whisking after each addition (you're building the sauce here so it's good to pause and let things thicken before the next addition). For the final thickening of the sauce, bring to a simmer for a few minutes and continue to whisk until the mixture thickens enough to easily coat the back of a spoon. Remove from heat and stir in the garlic, salt, and gruyere cheese.

3. Pour the sauce over the green beans. Cover with foil and bake for 25 minutes. Uncover, and bake for another 15 minutes. Give the green beans a quick toss to get them nice and coated in the sauce. Wipe down the edges of the casserole dish. Then, top with fried onions and bake for another 5 minutes. Let stand for

5-10 minutes to let the sauce settle into all its silky-smooth glory.

Prep Time: 25 Minutes

Cook Time: 1hrs 10 Minutes

Servings: 8

Ingredients

- 1 pound bacon, cut into small pieces
- 1/2 onion, finely chopped
- 1 clove garlic, minced
- 2/3 cup cornmeal
- 2/3 cup flour
- 1/4 cup sugar
- 1 tablespoon baking powder
- 1/2 teaspoon salt
- 1 cup sour cream
- 1/2 cup butter, melted
- 1 egg
- one 15-ounce can corn, drained
- one 15-ounce can cream-style corn
- 1 1/2 cups sharp white cheddar
- Chopped chives

Instructions

1. Preheat the oven to 350 degrees. In a pan over medium heat, fry the bacon pieces until crispy. Remove from the pan, but leave some of the bacon grease to sauté the onions. Add the onions and a sprinkle of salt to the pan and cook until softened. Add in the garlic and cook for another minute. Take the pan off the heat. Chop the bacon into bits.

2. In a bowl, combine the cornmeal, flour, sugar, baking powder, and salt. In a separate bowl, whisk the sour cream, butter, and egg until smooth. Then, stir in the corn, cream corn, the onion mixture, half of the bacon. Add in the dry ingredients, and stir until just combined.

3. Pour into a greased casserole dish. Bake for 35 minutes. Remove from the oven and top with the cheese and remaining bacon. Bake for another 5 minutes. Sprinkle chopped chives over the top.

Prep Time: 25 Minutes

Cook Time: 30 Minutes

Servings: 8

Ingredients

- 8 slices bacon (I find that thin bacon works better)
- 16 dates
- 4 ounces goat cheese
- toothpicks

Instructions

1. Preheat the oven to 350 degrees Fahrenheit. Slice the dates lengthwise on one side to create an opening. Remove the pit.
2. Using a spoon, stuff a small amount of goat cheese into the cavity of each date and press the sides together to close.
3. Cut the bacon slices in half. Wrap each date with a slice of bacon and secure with a toothpick.

4. Arrange evenly on a baking sheet with raised edges (otherwise grease will get everywhere) and bake for 10 minutes. Remove the dates and use the toothpick to turn each one so it's laying on its side. Bake for another 5-8 minutes, until browned to your liking, and turn the dates to the other side and repeat. Remove from the oven, place on a paper towel lined plate, and let stand for 5 minutes before serving.

9 798399 957852